SURVIVING
AIDS

SURVIVING
AIDS

THE MANY STORIES OF SURVIVAL IN OUR TWENTY-SIX YEAR BATTLE AGAINST HIV/AIDS

DAVID W. DRIVER

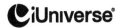

SURVIVING AIDS
The Many Stories of Survival in Our Twenty-
Six Year Battle Against HIV/AIDS

iUniverse books may be ordered through booksellers or by contacting:

iUniverse
1663 Liberty Drive
Bloomington, IN 47403
www.iuniverse.com
1-800-Authors (1-800-288-4677)

ISBN: 978-1-5320-0770-5 (sc)
ISBN: 978-1-5320-0771-2 (hc)
ISBN: 978-1-5320-0717-0 (e)

Library of Congress Control Number: 2016917584

Print information available on the last page.

iUniverse rev. date: 10/28/2016

Jordyn and I would like to dedicate this book to all of the family members who have supported us for the past 26 years. They have supported us in so many ways that you could never count them up. Those hero's being Versiellen my Mother, Johanna my sister, DJ my brother-in-law, Michelle my sister and Steve my brother-in-law.

We would also like to dedicate this book to the thousands of people who have kept Jordyn's prayer pin for all of these years to pray for Jordyn's continued good health.

PREFACE

Inside this book you will find different snapshots of time from our 26 year battle against the virus known as HIV/AIDS. The stories in this book span from the very beginning of our journey battling the virus. This also happened to be the beginning of the world wide battle against HIV/AIDS. At this terrible point in time there was very little hope as well as very little in choices medications.

As our war against this virus carried on there have been many different stories written about different snapshots in time, some that clearly let you look right inside the medical issues we faced. The others stories may at sometimes seem like they are out of place, but what you have to understand is when the AIDS virus enters your life it effects every aspect of your world.

In the beginning, this book was written to help our friends understand what was going on in our world. Because no matter how close you may think you are you can never really know what it's like. The only true way to know this monster is to stand eye to eye in the trenches of battle.

What follows next is a little poem I wrote to help outsiders understand the crazy world we were living in.

AIDS TO YOU, AIDS TO ME.

For you AIDS is Acquired Immune Deficiency Syndrome. Something you may fear.

For us AIDS is all that I do to survive. This is our daily challenge.

AIDS to you? Probably something that may sit in the back of your mind that you really don't want to think about much.

AIDS for us? Well, this is a whole different animal. For us it is the day in and day out, hour by hour, minute by minute challenge to do all the right things. For to survive this monster is a complex task of making all the right moves.

For you it's a life that hopefully you will never really know, because no matter how close you may get to it you, will never truly know this monster we call AIDS.

For us it's a complex journey of making all the right choices: Get the right doctor, take the right medicine and stay on course watching all that we do. For to stay alive in this game there is very little room for error.

AIDS to us is trying so hard to survive it, that we don't know what we are missing. You spend most of your time trying to catch up from all that you missed out on when you were distracted, trying not to die. I will tell you, that's one hell of a challenge.

AIDS to you, well it could be that you are in the dark. Maybe too afraid to be informed. Maybe too scared to get tested. These are the two biggest mistakes a person can make. Don't be afraid - Be informed.

AIDS for us has become our personal mission of being a gateway of information for those of you who have the need to ask and learn. Our mission is to also let people know that life is good in spite of all the chaos AIDS brings into our lives. That we have learned to laugh in the face of the unknown. To be positive no matter what may be challenging to us on any given day. For this is how we make it in our little world.

AIDS for you, it could become a new mission to help someone you don't even know, just because they might really need your help, but will never ask.

CONTENTS

CHAPTER 1

YEAR ONE: THE LEARNING CURVE

A GIFT OF TIME

A Gift of Time, was written so that our friends
could know and understand the situation
that our family was facing

We are so grateful for the emotional support from the
church, the church members and our friends have given us...
For all the prayer lists that we are on along with all the other
countless things that people have done to help us.

In this time of tearful tragedy, our hearts have been repeatedly uplifted by the goodness and kindness of people. It is so very IMPORANT for everyone to know about this illness. For this is no longer a disease that happens to other people.

These letters were written to give some facts that we were, not always strong enough to repeat over and over. That does not mean that we do not want to talk about these things. Only that sometimes we can and sometimes we cannot. One rule that we adopted very early on is that crying is O.K.

So here begins the story of Kari-Ann, David and Jordyn. Kari-Ann and Jordyn had always had an unusual amount of medical problems for such healthy looking young ladies.

In the late summer of 1989 I married my beautiful Kari-Ann, one might described her as the real Western woman, strong in spirit and frame... The type of woman you would see walking beside the covered wagon.

In March of 1993 Kari-Ann began to have numbness in her right hand, fingers and in her mouth. The numbness quickly spread to her whole right arm. She was referred to a neurologist. Prior to that appointment blood test were taken. On June 15 Karri-Ann was forced to go to the doctors alone due to the fact that I had just started a new job that very day.

On this day, Kari-Ann learned for the second time that she was HIV-positive. Not going with her to that appointment is one of the biggest regrets I truly hold onto to this day. In life making money is making life and you just have to do what you have to do when you're the breadwinner weather you like it or not. On hearing this news, tests were ordered for Jordyn and I.

Right after hearing this devastating news we were off to Colorado to attend my sister Johanna's wedding. Not telling Johanna or anyone else the bad news, thinking it would bring sorrow to the festivities. David shared this bad news only with his sister, Michelle. Kari-Ann was in tremendous pain from the spinal tap she received right before we left town. The exhaustion of the long automobile trip, and emotional bombshell was pretty overwhelming, but she handled it like a true champ attending the wedding ceremony, dancing a few slow songs and in general slowly but surely, taking part in all the events associated with a big family wedding. When we returned to Las Vegas, it was off to see the H.I.V/A.I.D.S. specialist to confirm that not only was Kari-Ann HIV positive, but that she was also in a state of full-blown A.I.D.S., with the T-cell count of 38. Mercifully, my test was negative. Our ongoing nightmare was that Jordyn's test was positive. Jordyn was given a life expectancy of 2 to 9 years. We expected nothing less than a miracle for Jordyn. We are all doing a lot of praying. We feel sure that you will join us.

The most shocking thing about Kari-Ann's being positive for A.I.D.S. was that blood tests were required in California before we were married. Why her condition was not found at the time made for a very large and open question that was never really answered.

Things happened so quickly, it's hard to remember how it all fit into such a short period of time. Immediately upon their return to Vegas, Jordyn was operated on for a gland infection. When she got out of the hospital, Kari-Ann traded places with her. Kari-Ann had contracted PCP, a type of pneumonia which is particular to AIDS patients. It is not contagious but never completely heals in AIDS patients. It is most often the cause of death in AIDS patients. Kari-Ann's condition deteriorated at an unbelievable rate. She also suffered from PML. PML is a disease that causes swelling around your brain stem. As the swelling increases it begins to cut off bodily functions one at a time. By August she could no longer dance, she could no longer walk or feed herself. She had also lost most of the power of speech. My Mom, Versiellen, had been planning to come in December too spend the year in Vegas to play with my granddaughter and give us a break. When Kari-Ann first got sick, we thought she had a minor stroke.... So my Mom had already started moving the date closer.

On August 9, I phoned my Mom in Florida. I said "Mom when I took Karri Ann to the doctor's office today, she said to me, "I know I'm going to die. I know it's going to be very soon. I'm okay with that but don't let them put me in a hospital..... Please don't let them take me away".

Since my Mom's arrival on August 11, she and I have wadded through a lot of problems. We became a part of a wonderful organization known as Hospice. They help keep patients at home and in a state of dignity. Her life expectancy was changed to six months.

On October 26 I had the heart rendering task of explaining to my little daughter that mommy had gone to live in the sky.

Kari-Ann was able to have her last wish. We were able to care for her at home which was so important to her. She died at home in dignity and peace.

Jordyn is enjoying the best health she has ever had, that's due to proper medical treatment. She is taking the only available H.I.V. medicine called AZT. In September she had surgery to install a port-ta-cath. It is like a two way valve in the blood vessel. Through the port they can take blood and give IV treatment. Once a month she gets a gamma globulin treatment to boost her immune system. This process takes about five hours. Trust me, she is one brave little girl.

If you see her looking up at the sky with her little lips moving. Just know she is having a talk with her mom. And she is okay with that right now.

About my Mom and I...well I'm very proud of my Mom. We do stress out at times as would be expected, but somehow we have found ways to process the challenges and sorrows in our little world. Together we put together mountains of care, tenderness, kindness and love to make this new little family unit work.

As for me, those of you who know me, know that I was always a little crazy and that hasn't changed. God gave us a "GIFT OF TIME". We think, we used it well with Kari-Ann. Our objective is to keep using that time wisely and joyfully. In Jordyn We have a grand task facing us.

Reverend Schuler once said, "You have a right to be happy in spite of your problems." That is what we have tried to do and will continue to do.

SHOCK WAVE

April 26, 1994

It hard to believe that it has been seven months. Seven months since the love of my life lost her battle against A.I.D.S. Here is the tale of how this shocking story unfolded.

To give you a little background, let's start at the beginning for this very special couple. They met, fell in love, got pregnant and got married. They were not the perfect couple in the beginning. There were numerous arguments in the beginning. This young couple had rules, like no fight ended without reaching a mutual understanding. As time went on, there was soon a new life, Jordyn. A family unit was formed. What a special time this was for the young couple. The addition of Jordyn brought a whole new reason for being alive, a whole new meaning and purpose to work for. As time rolled on, we began to really become one as a couple. We began to grow and learn together. This family learned how to survive some tough hardships. Learned how to scratch and claw in order to stay above water. Then in the month of March, Kari-Ann started having some minor medical problems. First it was in a numbness in her right hand. She did not pay much attention to it, thinking it would go away. Then suddenly she was having difficulty speaking. After a lot of prodding from me, Kari-Ann finally went to see her doctor. The doctor had various blood test taken, including a test for the HIV virus. Meanwhile, Kari-Ann was referred to a neurologist. While at her first neurology appointment, she learned the horrible news that she was HIV-positive, (This was June 15, 1994). I'll tell you to hear that kind of news is just unreal. You feel like you're in a time warp or something. I'm not really sure how I felt at the time, I guess I was really scared.

At first we thought that to be HIV positive was a bad thing, but we also thought, "Hey we can fight this". Little did we know what we were in for? While we were at the doctor's office Kari-Ann had to have a spinal tap.

"No big deal they said," RULE NUMBER ONE: DO NOT TRUST THE DOCTORS.

Kari Ann had her spinal tap and off we went to my sister Johanna's wedding in Colorado. No one really knew what a trooper Kari-Ann was, she was in a great deal of pain the entire weekend. Since it was Johanna's wedding, we decided not to tell anyone the news not wanting to spoil Johanna's big day. Upon arrival in Colorado I couldn't stand to hold it all in. I had to say something because it was really killing me. I finally told Michelle, my other sister, what was making me so crazy. Needless to say, she was mortified but kept my confidence.

Well from here on it starts getting really crazy. Once we were back home from the wedding, our little Jordyn had develop small bumps on her neck. After consulting with a doctor, she had surgery to remove them. So Jordyn spent three days in the hospital. While we were at the doctor's office, Jordan and I were tested for HIV virus. A couple days later I started working at a new job. Being the new kid on the block, I could not take time off to go to the second doctor's appointment with Kari-Ann and boy I wish I'd gone! As I turned in the apartment complex, I saw Kari-Ann sitting out front of our apartment. I knew that the second test was positive as well. I do not think I will ever get that scene out of my mind as long as I live, poor Kari-Ann. For me there was nothing I could say, there was no way for me to make her laugh. Oh my God, what do we do?

Things began to move faster now. Together Kari-Ann, Val, Karri Ann's sister, and I went to see the AIDS specialist, Dr. Cade. What a day to remember! I don't really know what made me ask the questions I asked, but I just had to know. For the first time in my life I felt like a real adult. Being a so-called head of household, I had to know what I was really dealing with. I would have given anything to not be that person, but I guess sometimes you are just chosen. It is hard to remember, once in a while, some of the events. But I know I will never forget the way I felt when I asked Dr. cade "how will we know when the HIV virus turns into AIDS?" His reply was that Kari-Ann was already in the AIDS classification. To me that was a tremendous shockwave. We went from fighting the HIV virus to fighting AIDS on the same day. Big difference! Once again I have to say that everything happened so fast some of the facts might be kind of foggy.

Even with all the terrible news we went home prepared to do battle. That was on Monday. Little did we know what would lie ahead? Along comes Friday like usual I get up to go for work, get my stuff ready, I am almost out the door when I go back to kiss Kari-Ann good-bye and noticed that she had a little fever. At the time I thought nothing of it. However, after I go to work I started to think about that fever and thought it could be a big problem. So I went home. Once I got home Kari-Ann's fever had subsided and I thought all was well. You know that a normal person with a fever is nothing special. This is not so for an AIDS patient. Soon the fever returned and I began to worry again. So off to urgent care we went. After threatening all the people involved, they finally admitted

Karri Ann. One thing led to another and soon she was in the hospital with pneumonia (the killer of AIDS patients. I thought). I was wrong. Kari-Ann fought back and beat that pneumonia and got to go home. Little did we know what a bad turn the disease would take?

People will never really know the speed with which this disease can strike. For Kari-Ann it was lightning fast. Within six or seven days she went from being able to walk and talk to hardly being able to sit up in bed. I knew things were really bad when Val came over to help and she broke out in tears upon seeing Kari-Ann's condition. From that time on Kari-Ann was confined to a wheelchair. It was time once again to see Dr. Cade. On the drive over to Dr. Cade's office I stopped and had a talk with Kari-Ann. I asked her what her wishes were. What do you want to do with the situation? I told her it was her life and whatever she wanted was what she would get. At this point Kari-Ann became the bravest person I have ever known when she said "David I know I'm going to die and I do not want to fight it, just let it happen, "she also said, please no more hospitals!" So we made it happen! We got a hospital bed from the union hall and designed a room for Kari- Ann's final days. Days later my mother Versiellen threw all her belongings into one bag and came to help me with Kari-Ann. From then on Kari-Ann had her ups and downs and I hope maybe even some happy days. As quick as it started it was over. October 25, 1994 she was in a tremendous amount of pain. The drugs I had access to did no good. We soon brought in the hospice nurse. She brought the real deal Morphine. Just minutes after the shot Kari Ann was at peace, no pain, no struggle.

On October 26, 1994 my mother called me at work. She said that the nurse had been by and said since Kari-Ann's body did not have to fight the pain anymore, she should probably be able to pass on in peace. Well as I drove home, I tried to take in everything so I could remember this day. I bought her rose's one last time. A couple hours after I was home, she finally slipped away. No more pain, no more struggle, she was finally done.

As for the new family unit, Jordyn, Versiellen and David, that's another story itself.

WHY?

Why??? That is the big question I ask. Why did God have to take the life away from a person that had so much to give?

Why does God impose such horrible illnesses on little innocent children? What is the purpose for making these children suffer? Although, I would have to say He, at least gives these special children an unbelievable amount of cheer and courage. I have watched these little kids play at school and wonder if they know as I do that they are so special.

I remember the first day I picked Jordyn up from Reach Out, a special day care for kids with HIV/AIDS, I looked around and saw all these beautiful children and wondered how long I would see them here.

You know it's not just the HIV kids though. I remember when Jordyn went to the hospital to have her Port-A-Cath put in. There was this little girl in the next bed who had leukemia. What a terrible thing to have to go through chemotherapy! I thought this poor little girl lost all her hair, but when asked about her hair her only response was, "well at least I don't have to brush it anymore". What a beautiful silver lining that little girl found all on her own.

The hardest part of all this is who do you trust with the life of your little girl? With HIV being so new to this world,

I sometimes think that the doctors don't really know what to do. It seems that they are following this formula and they have blinders on. Therefore, they may not be open to new ideas that might be of extreme importance.

Here I am, a single father that has to make basically life and death choices for my daughter. Whether I choose AZT or go the natural route. It is a gamble with my daughter's life. My gut feeling is to take her off all this mass amounts of chemicals. Something inside me tells me AZT is wrong, but there is that chance my gut feeling is wrong. What a perplexing position to be in. You get all the advice you can from everybody you know, but in the end it all boils down to the making the decision.

WHAT TO DO?

WHO TO BELIEVE?

WHO DO YOU TRUST?

In my life, I have been in a lot of difficult situations, but NOTHING has prepared me for the choices I have to make now. The really terrible part of this is that I can make all the right calls, but still lose my LITTLE GIRL.

To watch this little girl over the past four years has been nothing but pure pleasure for me. I try not to think about the future very much. Although, it is hard not to have dreams for your child.

All my life I have wanted to be a Daddy. I don't know how a parent could choose not to be a part of their child's life. I remember when Jordyn was first born, I felt really weird, kind of left out. I did not get that overwhelming feeling that I thought I would get. I really felt left out. However, as time went on that feeling hit me like a ton of bricks. Having Jordyn gave my whole life purpose. It made going to work more enjoyable. Finally my life had a real purpose to raise my little girl. What a turn on it was. When Jordyn says to me, "Daddy you make me so happy," that is the greatest feeling in the world.

Getting back to Kari-Ann. I really do not think anybody really knew Kari-Ann the way I did. She was the first girl who did something nice for me, right out of the blue for no reason at all. Kari-Ann helped me grow in a lot of ways, that I did not know I could grow. She had the guts to take me head-on and help me change a lot of my bad habits, and boy did we fight. Our rule was that our fights always went in the direction of solving the problem not eluding it. I remember when I knew I was going to be with her forever. It was when we had our first big fight! I was so mad I wanted to kill her, but at the same time I knew she already had won my heart. I think Kari-Ann and I would have been married forever. We were both really committed to our marriage. We had rules. 1) Never fight over money. 2) Always argue to the conclusion. 3) Never go to bed mad at each other. I'm really going to miss Kari-Ann forever and ever….. She was my best friend and pal. She had her faults, but she was always moving in a positive direction of growth. There were a lot of things she was afraid to do. But with a little pushing from me at the right time she would overcome some of her major obstacles. We were good for each other, in that we pushed each other to grow. Kari-Ann had talents no one could match. I think when she was born, God gave her a gift to make things and people beautiful. She had a big heart, and I loved her for that.

THE NEW HOUSE

Well tonight is the first night in the new house. It is such a great feeling to finally have a real home. I feel really lucky to be able to have this wonderful home. You know though, sometimes I feel really guilty about having this house without Kari-Ann. We worked so hard to save our money, and we did without so that we could reach this great achievement. I hope that wherever Kari-Ann is, she can get a little happiness knowing that it has finally happened.

We put up with the no money years together. That is probably the hardest part of everything that has happened. Not so much that she had to go, which in itself was probably the hardest thing to be a witness to, but what really brings me down, is that now the money is good, and all these great things are happening in my life and she's not here. It's just not the same dream without her around.

I guess that's where they get the line life is not fair. I think that she would love this house. We could not have done it without her, because even in dying she kept giving.

"I love you, wherever you are, Kari-Ann."

SEVEN MONTHS

Well it's been seven months since Kari- Ann has passed away. I really thought, by this time, I would have started to get over her being gone, boy, was I wrong. One thing I've learned from all this is that you can never really know the feelings you are going to feel. It does not matter how prepared you think you are and I thought I really had it handled. You can never really know how you're going to react until that time comes.

The reactions and the emotions you go through are so totally different from what you expected. I don't think anyone can really know how much you can miss that one special person in your life. Kari-Ann and I were such great friends as well as lovers and married partners. I think the hardest thing for me to get over are the weekends. The weekends were a very big part of our lives. The time we spent together on the weekends was a special time for dreaming together about what we wanted to achieve in our lives. The weekends were almost always a special time. It was our time, when we would share our most special feelings. I really miss those special times.

What I would like to know is what to do with all those dreams that we shared. It is really hard for me to have any dreams for the future now. I know that it may sound close minded for me to think that way. I really have a hard time looking ahead because of all the complications that I now have to deal with.

On a different subject there is Kari-Ann's family. It has been very hard to be cordial to them. It seems that they have all written us off, as if we do not exist anymore. It is hard for me to understand since Kari-Ann's service why no one in the family has made an effort to see how Jordyn and I are doing. How do these people, who were family just turn their backs on us now? I cannot understand how one day we are family, and the next day it seems that we are strangers. When we did finally hear from one of the family members by phone, they seemed so sincere and caring while they were on the phone, but that is as far as it goes. That just seems to be their total level of involvement. Well I have to say that this is just their loss not to have Jordyn in their lives, is their biggest mistake.

ONE YEAR

As you know things have happened pretty fast. I am pretty sure it was around this time last year that our lives changed forever!

I guess with everything happening so fast it kind of puts you in a kind of haze mentally. I remember thinking that even though all of these bad things were happening I could deal with them and in time I would be able get over this tragedy. Little did I know just how long and hard it would be?

They say that getting a divorce is worse than when someone dies, but I say it's not. The big difference to me is that when someone is gone, you know all the things that they are missing out on. You really want them to be there to share things with you. You just know they can't be. This is in contrast to a divorce, where you cannot share that special moment or feeling with them, you know however, they are still alive and able to have their own special moments and feelings. A good example of this is when I took Jordyn to Leaps Bounds, I found myself thinking about Kari-Ann missing out on the fun. On the other hand, if we were divorced, she would still be able to enjoy the experience with her little girl. Maybe you can see why I seem to be off in the fog sometimes, it's really hard to separate my happy feelings from my sad ones.

Sometimes when I see my little Jordyn, it just makes me the happiest man on earth. I feel lucky be in her presence. However, other times I just see all the things her loving mother is missing and that really kills me. It is so hard to balance that emotional line. Hopefully, someday I'll only see the joy that Jordyn brings to me.

The hardest part of getting over all of this is seeing other families having fun together. I see them and I am happy for them. Then again I have mixed feelings because the thing I miss the most is having my family! My family is the most important thing in my life. I do not think I will ever have that again and it truly hurts me inside.

I wish God could take that lonely feeling away from me. How do you get over that incredible gap that is left in your life when you lose your best friend and lover? I do not want another one because I had the perfect one.

All I want to know is, what do I do now? Where do I go from here? And when will this all end? It has already been a long, long road.

"Please God, help me close the gap."

PANIC TIME!

You know what the hardest things about having a healthy child with the HIV virus, is the way you feel. Most of the time things go on pretty routinely as if everything is normal, well at least that's the way it looks on the outside. There is also the other side that I try to not think about, I try to block it out. The main thing I block out is the future, I know what can and will eventually happen. I am basically a positive person, but sometimes reality can hit you right square in the face. Boy does it hurt!!! So everything in life is going along just fine and then it happens, your little one hurts. It really doesn't matter what the element is, because they all scare the hell out of you. Any illness can be a killer in this world of HIV/AIDS.

This is the PANIC TIME!!! This is the time your mind starts working double time fighting within itself for control. One side is the positive side always saying that it's no big deal. The other side is the reality always trying to deal with the problem at hand.

What to do for her?

Who do you call?

How to feel? There's no real answer for this one.

It can really be a struggle to keep afloat in the panic time. Somehow you manage altogether for the sake of that very special one, your little girl.

Luckily, she will get well and life will get back to normal. That is until the next PANIC TIME!

A SPECIAL TIME

Well, it's Sunday morning and here I sit on the patio watching the most beautiful sight. It's not anything special, just my little Jordyn playing in the sandbox. Our life is so busy that we hardly have time for times like this. Just me and Jordyn. This is not to say that we do not spend time together, because we do. It's just that we are always on the go to somewhere or are doing something that keeps us busy. So I have to say that times like today are pretty special moments. When the special times do occur, I want to freeze them and stay right here on the patio forever. For right here and now there are no worries, no tears, and no fears, for right now we are just going to be pals and play. Right now, life is truly GRAND!

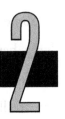

CHAPTER 2

THE NEVER ENDING BATTLE FOR LIFE

TWENTY ONE YEARS REMOVED

Well it's October 26 and it's really kind of funny how this day always creeps up on me. You would think that a day that changed your life forever would be a date that is engraved in your mind forever. Losing my Kari-Ann on this day October 26 1993, 21 years ago today was a day I surely thought I would never be able to overcome. You know in some ways it was easy to deal with because I had no choice. There was no going back that was for sure. Sitting here 21 years later and all alone in my adult world, it really makes me think about the days when I had a lover, that was also my best friend. You know when we were together, it was like a special world that no one got to see, except for the two of us. Kari-Ann had a beautiful smile that was so full of warmth and happiness, I surely miss that.

Sometimes I catch myself thinking about what if, but I always have to stop myself right away because that is a very dangerous game to play. If you value your sanity at all, you can never really let yourself go down that road. So instead I hold onto the select few really solid times that we spent together that will always make me smile. My most favorite day of all has to be the day we drove out to Lake Mead in one of the worst thunderstorms we had ever seen. The whole time we were driving, we just kept telling each other that when we made it there, we would have the whole lake to ourselves, because we were the only ones with enough faith to know it would be a special time for us and boy, were we right. We had so much fun just being with each other, not having to share our time with anyone else, just having the whole world to ourselves was amazing and was so special because it was just the two of us.

Yes it is 21 years later and a lot of time has passed, but no amount of time can ever make me forget my beautiful Kari-Ann

ARE WE REALLY GOING ANYWHERE?

You know for the past 6 months or so life has seemed to be in a weird kind of holding pattern. I am having a really hard time seeing down the road, or maybe it is because I am not seeing much down the road that interest me. It seems that day in and day out the things I am looking for in life are just not there. In a lot of ways it seems that all my hard work and dedication to being a great parent has left me all alone at the end of this journey. I guess my thoughts were that things would roll my way because I did what was right. Maybe in the end there really is no karma stored up for all of my doing what I knew was right. I'm really not asking for a whole lot friend. I just want somebody to notice, besides my family, I'm alive. Somebody that would take the time to look at who I am, and know I'm worth being around. Someone that would see the good person I try to be.

TOO MUCH!!

When do we get to coast? I mean I really think that at this point in our lives we have put up with enough crap that we've earned the right to coast a little. When is enough, enough? It seems like every day brings a new and different health issue. Some of these new issues have no real answer. I'm not asking for a miracle, I'm already over that. I would just be happy to see my little girl have a couple of months of good old normal boring life. I really just don't understand why we are forced to endure so many hardships.

Where is this notion of Karma? I mean in spite of all the hell we have lived through, we always try to overcome it with a smile and not let it change who we are or the way we treat others. I tell you some days it's just more than I can bear. It is really harder and harder to keep up a positive attitude when under the constant pressure of dealing with an illness that has no name, but has no problem inflicting its wrath day in, day out.

They say that the challenges in your life only make you stronger. Well that may be what they say. All I can tell you is it makes me feel pretty worn out. After all this time it just feels like we are in a very long tunnel, and it's very hard to see the light. It has been such a long time dealing with one crisis after another, that it gets harder and harder to find the silver lining. So I just try to make the days pass by as fast as possible, hoping that each day will end without issue. Just how long is one expected to carry on without a glimmer of hope? Could there be a solution on the horizon?

You know over the past 23 years of taking care of all these issues that seem to come my way, I have tried very hard to take it all in stride and not let it change who I am. I really don't want to be one of those people who thinks that everyone owes me for what I have been forced to live through. I have done it because it was the right thing to do, and I have very few regrets.

You know even with very few regrets, my mind likes to wander off, looking for the payback for all of my responsible choices. When my mind wanders off I think you know the world could do a little watching out for me. It seems only fair trade for all of the challenges that I have endured, that a little goodness could fall in my lap to let me know that it's not always an uphill battle. I just want to feel alive, connected to someone, who thinks about what would make David happy, and help ease some of this pain I have in this very lonely heart of mine. Just someone, outside of my family circle, who in their busy day stops to think, "I wonder how Dave is doing". Someone who would call me just to see how I was doing.

So world, here's your chance to step up and pay it forward to David Driver!!

HANDS TIED

Well this story starts off like this. I've been a single parent now 23 years and in all of that time I have always managed to find a way to make things work no matter what the obstacle. Maybe that's what makes what I'm about to tell you that much more aggravating. You see sometime around the year 2005 a monster with no real name started visiting my daughter. I call it the monster because after every conceivable test known to mankind the Doctors still couldn't put a finger on what was causing this pain. Not only did this monster decide to make her stomach its home. He decided to take control of our world in the form of intense pain. Little by little this monster started to take control of both of our worlds. In a very short period of time this little monster became a full-grown problem.

I guess the "hands tied" title comes from the fact that there is no real game plan in place. In the past years as a father of a terminally ill child, I have always managed to have some kind of game plan and would stick with it, and ride out the storm. So many times over the past few years I have sat and witnessed my daughter fight this monster and all I could do is stand there with my hands tied praying I could absorb her pain. There are no words to describe how defenseless it makes you feel to not be able to help your little girl. It just tears you in two.

You know in the past when the world would slap me in the face, I would respond by taking a deep breath and dive in to do what was needed to overcome the situation. Well it seems to me, that over the last three or four years there have been a lot of deep, deep breaths, but no solutions. Although I will never quit trying, one just has to ask how long can one hold out.

CHOOSE YOUR WAY

Well today was another one of those fork in the road days. Most days in life seem to be pretty programed in a way. We all have our things we do because it's what we do. As to what a normal day is, well that is up for review and also changes from person to person and day by day. For what seems to be a perfectly normal day to one person could possibly be the worst nightmare to another.

Over the past 23 years I have traveled through a lot of different opportunities of choice. You may be thinking what the hell is he talking about? Maybe life is finally taking its toll on him. So you don't have to worry about my sanity, I will try to explain what I've just come to understand. When I say I have lived through a lot of choices, what I'm really talking about are all the amazing things that a person can be put through and still somehow survive. I know from personal experience that when life comes at you hard and fast, trying to take you down, it is easy to feel like the world has focused in on you, and you think to yourself, why this always happened to me? I know I've spent a lot of time fighting those feelings, but sometimes those feelings get in no matter how hard I fight. It is at these times that we begin to travel through the choices of life. You know when those challenging

33

times in life come knocking on your door, it may not seem like a great opportunity in life, but whether we recognize it or not, it is.

After answering the door many times I have come to the conclusion that, it is an honor, in a way, when the world comes knocking. At these times in life we are given the opportunity to make choices in the ways we respond to life. It is at this time where we really get to see who we really are, and who we really want to be.

In every challenge that we face in life there are many choices for us, it is what we choose and how we move forward that determines who we really are. There are many paths to choose from. The path less traveled, or a path easily walked on with little or no resistance. The path that has little or no resistance is the path that lets us find blame for problems in everyone else, as well as a reason to avoid the real issues we should be facing. I guess there's nothing wrong with this path. It's a very simple way to go. On the other hand, taking the high road, although more difficult, is a path where we will learn how to deal with the challenges brought to us, as well as truly learn the lesson the world wants us to learn.

At many times when I had the opportunity to stand at the fork in the road, there were many times I really wanted to just run down the path of least resistance saying "what the hell no one really cares which way I go". I deserve the easy way to feel a little joy instead of struggle. As you take the few first steps down that easy street you hear that voice in the back of your head saying "this is not your path. Any joy you think you are feeling has no foundation to make you feel the way you feel when you take the higher road". So as easy as this road may seem, I turn it around and go down the road I know is right for me.

So in the end I would like to say "thank you to the powers that be for giving me the chance to choose my way. Always helping me be the person I know I want to be, even if sometimes I really wanted to just go the other way. Thank you for always challenging me to continue on my path".

GROUNDHOG DAY!

We've all seen the movie Groundhog Day. You know the movie with Bill Murray. Where he keeps having to relive Groundhog Day over and over again. Well that's kind of how I feel my life has been for far too long to remember. The only thing is that there's not much humor in my story.

For a long, long time now the same thing has been happening pretty much every day. Every morning my daughter wakes up feeling like shit and is in a lot of pain. Every morning I wake up and hope that when I ask my daughter how she feels, this will be the morning she says, "I feel great, the pain has gone away". It's just like the movie no matter how hard I pray and wish that the answers to my questions would have a different answer- the answer being, no pain, that just doesn't happen. You know what the real crazy thing is about all of this, is that before this monster came into her life, she was already in the battle for life, a battle against HIV and AIDS. Long before this monster came into our lives we lived through, still are living through, the ongoing battle with AIDS. In our battle with AIDS we lost Jordyn's Mother and my best friend Kari-Ann. Living through those years I never thought there would be something that would come along that would put AIDS in the backseat. Although dealing with AIDS was and is scary at times, at least there were many days when my daughter never cried out in pain like she does now.

So just like in the movie Groundhog Day we have tried so many new approaches to overcome this monster that I'm running out of things to say to my daughter. I'm pretty sure she is getting tired of me telling her that this is the year it's all going to change. I really don't want to say that we have given up, but there's only so many times you can wake up to the same old story, it's difficult to have bright hopes for the day.

STAYING POSITIVE

Well here is another day whether we want it or not. You know sometimes it seems like greeting the new day is the scariest thing to do. I'm just so tired of day after day waking up alone and being alone. No matter how well I treat the people in my life, it seems like trying to have some friends is a losing battle. I try so hard to show the people in my life how important they are to me and always try to be there for them when I can. It really seems like it's not a two-way street. How one person can put out so much love and kindness, but feel so alone in the world at the end of the day. I can't even remember the last time I had a real smile on my face. I try so hard to stay positive in spite of my world, but that task seems to get harder every day. I will keep trying, it's like I have said many times "I'm just too stupid to quit trying because I know I deserve a better life than the one I am living".

THE PRIVATE BATTLE

There is a life that goes on that most people do not see from the outside. It is the battle we fight almost every day. A battle of mind and heart. When it comes to Jordyn's life, it is a complicated two edge sword for my family and me. On one side of the sword represents my family and me. This side of the sword is used every day, it's the constant care we have to manage day in and day out. We all strive every day to make sure Jordyn has all the proper diet, medicine and support she needs to stay alive. Then there is the other side of the sword. This side represents the unexpected things that come along. In the HIV world this can be many things. There are no simple problems in Jordyn's life when it comes to her health issues. All things have to be watched with a careful eye.

There is the part of Jordyn's life that outsiders never see. In Jordyn's life even the smallest things can become much bigger problems. You see every day can bring some new challenge for us. A simple stomachache for most kids turns into a crisis for us. Just when I start to feel that what we are going through is no big deal, along comes a call from the doctor. As I answer the phone one side my mind instantly goes into a state of panic, while the other side of my fights to stay cool, calm and collected. On the really special days the whole brain just tries to run away from home. As a parent I can't let my mind go crazy until I have all the facts, but it's that small moment in time right before I pick up the phone to call the doctor that seems like an eternity. In that small amount of time part of me wants to freak out and worry, all the while the other side of me knows I have to stay strong for my daughter and my family.

Sometimes I wonder if something is wrong with me when I don't worry enough. Have I been in this battle so long that I have become numb to all of this? I always try to stay on the positive side of life, but sometimes I just wish God would look down and see that my little girl has been through enough, and know that it's time for a break. We are still waiting for that to happen.

TIME SERVED

What the hell do we have to do to get the sentence to hell reduced for good behavior? I just don't understand how long my daughter has, to be dragged through the hell she has been living through for almost 7 years now. She has endured this monster inside her body, mostly with a good attitude and a positive outlook. She has never once lashed out in anger at the world for what she has had to go through. For the most part she has sat quietly and prayed for the pain to subside. Time and time again she has listened to me tell her to hang in there and don't give in. We will beat this, something will happen just have faith. She for the most part has done all that has been asked of her.

So where is the light at the end of the tunnel that we have worked so long for? It seems like every time we think we can see it, we are fooled and have to start down a new path. I cannot even count the number of paths I have asked my daughter to walk down to only find another dead end. How many times can I expect her to have faith in what I'm telling her? How many times can I sell myself about the latest plan I have dreamed up? Hopefully together we can keep each other from giving in. I swear I will never give up on her, but lately the challenge has been huge and very costly to, my mind and body.

THE PRICE OF A.I.D.S.

You know there has been millions of dollars raise in the name of AIDS, and that in turn has paved the way for many advances in medicine to help the unfortunate ones who have this disease. For they are the ones that have paid the unseen price of AIDS. What I mean by the price of AIDS is the costs of AIDS, which very few see. Beyond the medical bills is the personal cost that adds up over the years of fighting this monster. Most of the time you're so grateful that you and your loved one are doing well you don't dare tempt fate by thinking you have the right to be upset that your original life or dreams that you used to have are all but a distant memory. Let alone having any new dreams other than the dreams of you and your loved one's living a long life, because you have learned by now that any other dreams you may be silly enough to dream are crushed under the weight of the price of AIDS.

When on the battlefield of AIDS you have no time to see what has happened to your life. Your too busy going to doctors and hospital appointments as well as hundreds of phone calls keeping up on the people that are supposed to take care of her. For without your eternal vigilance your healthcare seems to just stagnate. So while you're doing all of this stuff, it never even dawns on you that your original life and its dreams fell by wayside. Simple things like going to high school football games, having a boyfriend, or being invited anywhere by your classmates. That's right - the other big price of AIDS is not having friends. You see a lot of your peers mean well in the beginning trying to be there for you, but as time goes on people seem to disappear no matter how good a friend they were in the beginning.

You see behind closed doors people start to realize for one reason or another they really don't want to be involved in a world that has the word AIDS in it. No matter how well their intentions were in the beginning, sooner or later this issue comes to head and that's when you lose another person in your life. As I look back over the last 23 years of living in the world of AIDS I have seen many, many good friends just disappear, no matter how hard I tried to be a good friend it just doesn't do any good, they are just gone. I guess I cannot blame them because when I look at my world from their point of view I probably would not want to be here either.

In the end I want to say that I tried to look on the positive side of life, trying not to think about the things I have lost to the AIDS virus, but to think about all I have learned on this journey.

CHAPTER 3

WORDS OF WISDOM
FOUND ON THE BATTLE GROUND

THE PRICE OF HONESTY

You might be wondering right now what in the hell is this guy talking about, it doesn't cost me anything to be honest. Well my answer to that is, it all depends on the people you are supposed to be honest with, and how being honest can cost you in ways you may never even stopped to think about. You see the people that make up our relationships and families they can be some of the most costly people in our lives. Most times we don't see them coming.

Here is how the tab starts to build. Everybody will want to tell you that being open and upfront about all the things going on in our lives is the way you should be. They will tell you that not telling them everything about the things that go on in your life is like telling a lie. So in the pursuit of trying to be a good person, we go along with the whole idea that our lives are an open book for all to read. Now this should be all right if the people that surrounded our lives would read the book with an open mind and heart. The real truth of the matter is that most of these people don't even take the time to crack open the book of our lives, let alone really read the story to see the things from all sides. It seems like there are a lot of people out there that are selling good intentions upfront, but lack the ability to really do what's right in the end.

So many times I've heard people tell me that withholding the truth is not right, so once again you try to do what you think is right. After you do your part by being totally open you start to realize how painful this can be sometimes. In most cases the people on the other side will take advantage of your uses very vulnerable times of your life to gain control of you by imposing their thoughts on how wrong you are and how right they think their line of thinking is. At a time in life where no one could be harder on you than you have already have been on yourself. Many people use this time to gain control by making you feel like you're less of a person because of the situation you're in. Very rarely do you have someone that remains the same person you used to know before this all started. They tell you to be honest and when you do, they take this time to take your honesty and use it like a club to beat you down, instead of trying to lift you up. Even when you could be totally in the right, no one tries to see that at all. You know the stress of dealing with your problems is big enough without someone else loading on the guilt complex. Seems like they get so caught up in creating a path to themselves, like what you are going through is affecting them just as bad even though they are not anywhere near the flame.

I guess this is why we learn how to not just open the top of our head for the whole world to look in. Sometimes we hold back because there is so much pressure on us from the assumptions of the people we are trying to face. Before we can admit our wrongdoing we are tried and hung out to dry by the people who said they would be there for us. Why is it that people think that because they want to help you that gives them the right to take over your life watching every step you take and telling you how to take those steps? Why can't people just help with what you really need and not what they want to force on you? In the end this becomes the most painful thing in the world because you want to feel grateful for their help, but their help is really just contributing to the problem in the end. Instead of your friends defusing the problem, they add gas to the fire in the end, by belittling you and the person you are trying to be. A true friend should just help you with the ingredients for the meal and not try to control kitchen.

MEN WITHOUT PANTS

Really who is raising all these men without pants? What I mean by this is that there seems to be a whole lot of male human beings walking around without their balls. I'm not talking about some of the married man in this world. What I'm talking about is all of these posers that stand around all day telling anyone who will listen to them what a man they are. I personally have known a few of these poser. Let me explain. These so called men that talk a good game should all be wearing little dresses since they sure don't seem to have either their balls or their brains. You see I'm talking about these posers that when in the wrong will spin their story to the left and to the right, but never will they look you in the eye and say I'm sorry that's my bad. Not only do they spin out of control trying to save their ass they also start tearing the people who are around them down with lies and rumors that have so little merit it almost makes you laugh when you hear the giant tale of bullshit they are trying to sell the world. I just don't understand how they look themselves in the mirror. To recklessly throw out what could be damaging lies at the people that they have already damaged to begin with. You know I am by no means perfect in any way shape or form, but sometimes I feel like I'm one of the few men left on this planet that lives up to my word as well as not being afraid to say "I'm sorry" I mean don't these fools realize that the only one who believes their bullshit stories is themselves. You know I'm happy to be the guy who says I'm sorry, because then I can put that problem behind me after I have learned the lesson, it comes with making mistakes. How can you ever really grow as a person if we don't own up to all of our mistakes? From the minute we were born we make mistakes. This is how we learn to grow up a move forward. Why would anybody want to trap themselves in the endless circle of lies?

I don't know when things started to fall apart in this world, when it comes to truth and integrity because it's a sad state to be in. So do the world a favor, next time you feel you may be in the wrong, don't give into your greedy side of your consciousness, and look for someone to hang all the blame on. Take the high road put on your pants, pull them all the way up and then say, "Hey I'm sorry about that, and what can I do to fix it?" As scary as that scenario may seem, you will be surprised at what a good feeling it can bring you.

BEING SO BLIND

People are really funny sometimes in the way that they react to areas outside of their normal realm, but feel like they know it all. Why is it some people assume that because you asked them for help, it's a green light for them to take over your world, without even really being asked. The really bad thing is the way they start to treat you like a 10-year-old child who doesn't know how to handle himself. Just because you may need a little help, should this be a green flag that says please treat me like a child and tell me how to walk and talk. In a time where your insecurities are running higher than normal, they make matters worse by trying to take over making you feel more insecure in the process. Just because a person is having a bad time does not mean he forgot how to talk or to act. These people go so overboard trying to run your world that they don't even notice the way they are tearing you down mentally and physically.

Why it is that no one stops to ask you how they can help you. It's because there too busy trying to assume that they know what's best for you and that you're too dumb to figure things out on your own.

So the next time someone needs your help, why don't you do the both of you a favor and just ask them, "How can I help you."

HAPPINESS ON TRIAL

You know when you really think about it, our happiness seems to be on trial every day of our lives. What I'm trying to say is that no matter how good I may be, or you may be at being in a good place that makes us happy, there always seems to be some outside source trying to imprison our happiness. It's almost like the world gets jealous when it notices the glow that happiness brings to a person.

Why is it that two people in a relationship that love each other find a way to derail this wonderful bliss instead of being grateful that they are one of the lucky ones a to be in a loving relationship. They instead have to search for the small cracks in the wall. Now that wall could be hundred feet high and hundred feet wide with no other cracks at all, but they're so busy looking at that one crack that they miss seeing all the greatness of the rest of the wall. Why as humans do we always find it so easy to tear someone else down finding all of their cracks? Don't you think it would be a good idea to find and repair our own cracks before we look elsewhere? There is so much more joy building up our lives then there is spending time finding reasons why we should tear them down.

So if you are a person who likes to make a difference in

this world, let's all promise each other a very simple promise. Let's all promise to be builders of happiness no matter how hard it is. Let's be the ones that lift people up instead of tearing them down by searching for the small cracks. Because remember crack kills.

LIKE BALLOONS

I was thinking the other day that we are all like a bunch of balloons tied together at the amusement park. When bunched up we spend too much time whining to each other about all of our problems. Instead we should really be talking about the adventure that lies ahead of us when we are set free from each other. I think it would be a lot more fun to talk about the great adventures ahead of us, not wasting our time on a bunch whining. So let's all cheer each other on as we release the balloons!

RESPECTING THE LINE

You know when I was growing up, I was taught to respect the law as probably you were as well. Now I don't know about you but in my mind the things that I have seen and heard lately have really given me good reason to not trust these people that are supposed to be protecting me. Growing up I was taught there is a defining line. On one side of this line there is the good side where everyone is honest and upfront. On the other side of the line are the liars, the cheaters, and people who do just what they want no matter how it may affect others. At one time in this world the majority of the police force always seemed too lived on the good side of the line leading by example. What I would like to know is when it became acceptable practice for some of them to cross the line to do their job. When did it become all right for the police to act like the crooks by lying and misrepresenting themselves in order to catch the bad guy?

I mean I thought they trained and went to school to learn how to outsmart the bad guys instead of becoming one of them. How are we supposed trust and respect them when they are not respecting their own oath they took in the beginning? So now we live in a world where the cops don't have to respect our rights and are doing very little to protect our rights.

We have cops that don't even respect the laws they are supposed to be upholding. When was the last time you heard about a cop getting a speeding ticket or a DUI? No, they all belong to that special officers club, where they all scratch each other's backs. Where their motto is "I won't tell on you if you won't tell on me". Which means they feel no need to obey the laws they are forcing everyone else to obey. What happened to the adage of lead by example? How can we have any respect for them if they are not respecting themselves? What really scares me is where this is all going and how far are they willing to go in an effort to make an arrest? Just how far over that line are they going to go to prove their worth?

In the end I feel bad for those officers that do walk that line, because their good work gets tarnished by the actions of these officers that have no problem crossing the line.

WORDS OF ENCOURAGEMENT

You know the other day my sister, Michelle, called me up to ask if I could offer some words of encouragement to a friend of theirs who was having problems with his health.

You see after a bout with cancer that he managed to survive and thought all was behind him, only to find out that it had resurfaced. I guess my sister asked me to reach out to him because of all the hell Jordyn and I have managed to survive over the past 23 years.

It seemed to be a simple gesture to do, but as I sat down to write him, I started to look back on the hard times that I've have gone through to see if at any time there came letters of encouragement from anyone that was witness to our little world of horrors. Sad to say there were none, so I wrote some of my own.

Over the last 23 years I have seen many people come and go in our lives, many with good intentions in their heart. But at this point we are still pretty much here by ourselves. The strongest people we have in our lives have always been my Mom, Johanna and DJ. I can understand why many that have tried to help just couldn't hang in there with the battle we had to wage on a daily basis. It just seems that even when we have won a battle and things will calm down, inside that little victory lies a new bundle of fresh issues at our door. Why is it that my little girl has to live through a continued onslaught of physical pain as well as the mental battle day in and day out? I think that after all she has been forced to endure over the past 23 years since her diagnoses. It should be her turn to just coast down the road of life and be able to be a normal kid. I have never seen a person so happy to just be normal.

When will it be her turn!

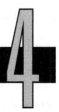

CHAPTER 4

THOUGHTS FROM MY HEAD

GASPING FOR AIR

Well it's just about a year now since the woman I came to love ran out of my life, leaving me gasping for air. Never in my life have I been so blindsided by someone that said they would love me forever, someone who said they wanted to spend the rest of their life with me. I will never understand how she could say all the things she said to me, including making a commitment to always be there for me and not run. Then without any real warning she just decides to end it all without even a discussion… just cut and run.

I really don't know how she can look herself in the mirror knowing the pain she put me through. I mean, here it is a year later and I'm still having a hard time staying afloat. I really don't know if I will ever be able to give myself 100% to another woman.

I still don't understand how I deserve to be treated the way she treated me in the end. I put all of my heart and soul into our relationship because of the bond I felt we had. What were all those long talks about us being together forever? We spent so much time talking about how we would be able to handle life's issues because we had each other and together we can overcome any obstacle. Just makes me sick to my stomach to think that it was all just a waste of time. I mean was she just bullshitting me every time that we sat alone and talked about our future? We talk so much about how lucky we were to have the special bond between us. Then she just walks away without even letting me talk to her at all, leaving me totally in the dark. To throw it all away without putting up any kind of fight to stay together. I feel so cheated that my whole life has been torn apart without even the tiniest chance to work things out. How do you tear someone's heart out based on what you think might happen in the future. How do you run your life based on what ifs? I find it so hard to believe that she was so selfish. She had no place in her heart for me, and was she lying to me all along.

I waited so long for the right woman to come into my life. Why it had to all be some kind of very cruel joke in the end. It could have very well been a deadly joke if it were not for the fact that I have become used to very painful situations over the years. I mean how many heart stopping events can a person live through and want to continue to live on in such pain. Wasn't losing Kari-Ann painful enough, now we had to add in a daughter with HIV, then just as I was learning to stand again I lost the first girlfriend I managed to find. Then there's the real topper - ten years in hell dealing with a phantom stomach pain that no Doctor can diagnose. Really how much is enough.....

You know I don't want a miracle, or to win the lottery, I just want to have a life that doesn't call for nonstop crisis after crisis. It's all I can do to keep me on the positive flow, but I just think I'm running out of pressure to keep me flowing. It is really, really time for the world to get back to Dave, before it's too late.

Can somebody just please throw me a bone!

THE DISAPOINTING TIMES IN LIFE

You know as a general rule I really try to stay on the positive side of life always trying to find the silver lining. Trust me when I say that over the past 23 years I have had many opportunities to walk around with a dark cloud over my head and still found a way to laugh it off.

You know no matter how good I may have gotten at hitting a curveball of life, there will always be my Achilles' heel, and that is the friendships I have lost over the years and the lack of any answers as to why it seems like people I have been friends with don't seem to see any value in our friendship the way I do.

I mean you have to know someone for a long time building a friendship and one day you look up and they're not there and there is no real apparent reason. This is the time that the clock starts ticking way the minutes, hours and days and months maybe years that I spend trying to figure out how these people can just disappear from my life. I don't really know how I went from being this person's friend one day to someone they never talk to again. I have a real hard time not thinking about how they are doing and how do they have this ability to just disconnect from the world we shared, to a world where they don't even think about me anymore. I wish I could figure out what I do that drives them away from me.

BEING ME

Being me. What does that really mean, there's a lot of people I know that will tell me who I am and how I think and what I need to do to find a happier me. Now most of these people that have this great view of how I need to be & how I need to do this or I need to do that to find a happier me really have no clue what they are talking about.

How could they know what I really need? Most of them have never really taken the time to sit down and really listen to what I have to say? Most of the people that surround my life spend so much time telling me why I should be happy or grateful that there's no possible way they took any time to sit quietly and listen to the thoughts that cloud my mind.

You know over the past 23 years there have been many nights spent alone with only me and my thoughts. On most of those nights where loneliness really tries to take control of my mind, this is a time where I really dig in and refuse to let the loneliness tear me down. Over the past 23 years I've used every tool in the box to keep myself in a place to remain in control of my mind that really just wants to let go and run like crazy. If one was to look back at the past 23 years and see all of the challenges thrown down at my feet, they would first think wow! Can it be possible, no one should have to live through that much shit?

Then their second thought would be, he must be making some of it up, because no one can live through all that and still be somewhat normal.

The third thought is that he's got to be hiding the real him and we need to help him by telling him all the things we think are best for him. Telling him that he really doesn't understand his own life. What's really funny is that these people are going to tell me how to survive a world they have no clue about. It's almost like a child telling a World War II veteran what it was really like on D-Day and how he should just get over it.

Then the real kicker is after all of their misguided advice they will leave and go home to their wife or girlfriend and leave me alone with my thoughts one more time. Don't get me wrong I know these people mean well, but if they took their good intentions just a little further maybe they would realize that what they should really be doing is take the time to listen to that person in need to find out what they really need, and not what you thought they needed.

Being alone without a partner to share the weight of living has been the hardest part. The thing is a partner that is in the trenches with you day in and day out is really the only one that can help you deal with your battles. When you go outside your world to vent your frustration, you end up running into someone who thinks they have all the answers and will tell you so and no matter how many times you try to get things off your chest, they're just so focused on telling you what they think is right. They won't let you just vent. Which in the end just magnifies your original nightmare. So if you really want to be that person to help to someone you know who is living in a world of hell, do the easiest thing you can do, just sit calmly and listen to them, Because this is what they really need. Most of the time after they have blown off a little steam and their head has cleared the solution to their problem has been there all the time and was only hidden by the steam built up in their head.

All they ever really needed is that special person to come along and say, "Hey man just let it out. I'm here to listen and not to try to solve your problems. I'm just here to catch you if you fall and help you get back on your feet".

Sometimes that can be the hardest thing to do!

ALONE IN THE ROOM

Well this is a place where a parent never really wants to be, it's a place I have been all too many times. It's a place where you're really are not alone because your child is sleeping just 5 feet away from you. Still you are so very alone. You see this room you and your child are in is a room where you will most likely share every emotion you can think of. In this room you will see your child become the bravest and the most terrified person you have ever known.

This is your child's hospital room. The way you end up alone in the room is that after all the blood has been drawn, and all the tests have been run, your child finally has found a way to fall asleep amongst all of the alarms going off. You are the only one left awake in the room. Now you are truly alone with you and your thoughts. At this point in time is where all of the day's events start fighting back in your mind giving you way too many things to contemplate for a body that is way too tired for this battle. It is at this time you really have to muster all of your strength and stand up to yourself and say don't start worrying about the things you think you know, and just deal with the things you know you know.

Sitting in that dark room is the toughest battle I have ever had to wage.

WHERE AM I REALY GOING?

You know for the last six months or so life has seemed to be in this weird kind of holding pattern. Seems like I'm not moving forward. This may be due to the fact that when I look down the road, I'm not seeing anything that draws me in. It seems like the day in and day out is just repeating itself.

Every day I wake up and hope this is the day where my life turns the corner heading toward some of the simple things I have really missed in my life, but by day's end I'm just as far away from those things.

You know raising a child alone is no ride in the park, then add in a lifetime of serious medical issues to make life a little more fun. Don't get me wrong, having my daughter in my life has been the greatest joy I could ever know. Just seems like after all the hard work I always thought there would be a little payback for hanging in there. I thought after dedicating my time to raise my daughter there would be some kind of life for me.

It's not like I did what I did because I thought there was a prize at the end of the journey. I did it because I love my daughter. Just never thought I would be so alone after my daughter had become an adult. I don't think I'm asking for a lot. It would just be nice to have someone in my life. Someone that could see the value in who I am and really wants to be part of my life. Someone that can see that after all I have been through I have managed to remain a person who just wants to be able to make that special woman happy and loved. I really don't think that's a lot to ask of this world that has challenged me so many times.

TRADING LOVE FOR PAIN

You know today started out like most days. You get up to start your day, but that is when this day also started to fall apart. Why is it when you love and care about someone they are so totally blind to the pain they can put you through? Why did they push you to a point to where you have to do things you would never normally want to do? How is it that you show your love and commitment to a child for 26 or so years to you raise them?

Then one day you feel like you have wasted your time because your child says things that you just can't believe and then they just walk away. Things that really send a parent into hyper overdrive thinking about where they are and what they are going to do. While I am not alone in this, hearing my daughter tell me she's done with me and the world and then leaves all of her belongings in a pile in the driveway of our home. Then she walks out of sight refusing to talk to me that pretty much tops the worst moments in my life. At that moment I felt like she traded her love for me for a pain I hope she will never know. I was out of my mind not knowing how to even breathe at the moment. In my heart I know we will get back to loving each other, but for the moment I moved on to the real fear that she really might do something stupid, which took me right back to the not being able to breathe thing. As panicked as I was at the time there was still the voice telling me she wouldn't go there. Wow! What a battle your own mind can have with itself at times like this. Trying not to worry and then worrying that if you don't worry that things could go wrong if you don't respect that possibility.

So I did the things all parents do, I called all of her friends to let them know what was going on so that maybe they could talk her down and let her know she was okay. Then came the anger over the way she treated me, totally without any love in her voice. Before ever saying the things she said to me that day she had to know how much pain those words would bring to me, but the words came hard and fast and full of pain just for me. As she walked away, I couldn't believe this is my girl. As much as it hurt me at the moment I knew in the back of my mind that these were only words thrown out in a time of battle, and not her true feelings, still they are hard to swallow. Guess that's like they always say, "You only hurt the ones you love."

Of course, this too passes, she is my little girl again.

IN A BIND

You know over the past 26 years I have faced a lot of challenges. I have always been able to overcome those challenges in one way or another. Right now I'm looking into one of the toughest situations that a person can be in. I'm in between a rock and hard place, me being in the "in between" part.

The really hard thing is this situation involves people I love dearly on both sides of this very serious issue. The issue being my daughter spending large amounts of my sister and brother-in-law's money. She used their credit card without permission and this is not her first offense. Needless to say they were and are pissed off and hurt that she has done this twice without taking accountability for her actions. So here I sit in between my daughter and my sister and brother-in-law trying to figure out how I can put the little family I have back together again.

On the one side I am in total agreement as to how wrong my daughter is and how lucky she is that they're not pressing charges.

To see how mad my sister was and to hear her calling my daughter a thief was tough to hear even if she is right. It turns my stomach inside out when I sit down and try to digest this problem. I know what she has done is huge and she must pay for her poor choices.

Then there is how Jordyn's mindset is after being sick her whole life with AIDS, and then adding in 10 years of severe stomach pains. She just doesn't have it in her mind the severity of the situation she has put herself in, as well as myself. Knowing my daughter as well as I do I understand where she is coming from even if she is misguided. We are meant to make mistakes so that we can learn from them.

The real problem is after all these years I think I'm just too worn down to be in the middle of someone who really wants to make their point and someone who is one step away from throwing in the towel. I know that DJ and Johanna are well within their rights to be mad and I feel their anguish.

I really want to be on both sides of this issue and that is what is killing me. A lot of people like to think they know what it's like to be in Jordyn shoes but they can only get a glimpse of what her hell is really like. Since she was diagnosed at the age of 3 she has gone to sleep many times afraid she will not be there in the morning. What does that do to her brain? On one side I really want to put it to her for putting me in the middle because it has been hell. On the other hand I can't even remember the last time I puked up my guts, and for Jordyn it's an everyday thing that she lives with. It's so hard to be the hammer when someone is throwing up every day. I really want to be tough but I'm just not that strong and it's only money in the end. I know that sounds really terrible and that's why I sit here with my soul turning itself inside and out all day thinking about this whole terrible mess.

I'm totally up for suggestions?

THIS TIME OF NIGHT

Well it happens every night for me. It's that time of night, the time to go to bed. It doesn't really matter what time it is, it's just the fact that once again I have to go to my room and be alone. This is the thing I really hate about my life, the constant loneliness. It feels like a prison term, like I have been sent to solitary confinement. I've tried many different ways to put an end to this sentence that I have been serving since my lovely Kari-Ann left this world. There have been a few short periods of relief, but those times just ended up causing me more pain and fear of trying to find someone to complement my life. Where's Karma when you really need her!

WHY DO I STAND ALONE!

Why do I stand alone? I asked myself this question way too many times; most times I get no real answer out of myself. When I stand back and look at who I am, I see a person who really tries to be a person of good character. I'm helpful to most people I knows. I'm a guy who really wants to be that friend that's there when you need him, someone you can count on. I try to be that guy who has really tried not to judge a person by how they look or where they come from. Someone that doesn't hold the past over someone's head it's their past is not who they are now. I myself as someone who really wants to love his friends for who they are but never gets that chance because it seems like for one reason or another people seem to just walk out of my life with little or no explanation as to why they just disappear. Which then makes me spend countless hours wondering what the hell he has to do to just have a good friend. I work very hard trying to be a standup guy, so why I'm I so alone at the end of the day?

You know I was raised to be the kind and warm hearted person who is responsible almost to a fault. How is it that these qualities seem to be a deterrent to having friends instead of them being a draw? It really drives me crazy to think of all the people I have met and have tried friends with, and yet here is another night sitting alone by myself. It's not like I don't like me because I do. I'm very proud of the man I am, I have no trouble looking in the mirror. I am a great guy, but I get tired of hanging out with me, I don't want you to think that I don't appreciate the people closest to me, namely my family. They are the soul of my backbone and I could not make it on this planet without them. It's just sometimes it would be nice to have someone outside of my circle of life to hang out with and talk about something other than my family circle.

In the end it seems like some cruel joke that the guy who wants to have friends the most, ends up being the loneliest guys on the planet.

53 AND EMPTY

So here I sit alone again, it's a scene that seems to be repeating itself no matter how much I hate the scene. The question I keep asking myself is, "what have I done so terrible to be sentenced to this solitary life that I can't seem to get out of". All of my life I've tried to do the right thing when it came to the people in my life.

I don't think there is another person that wanted to be accepted so badly by the people around him. I've always tried to be there for my friends when they needed some help in their lives.

How is it that I can put out so much positive energy and have it come back in such a negative way? I don't understand how being a good friend to everyone I know has turned out to be something that has come to haunt me. I mean after all these years to have no one you can call a friend is the emptiest feeling a person can have. To never have the phone ring for you in your own home is so very sad especially after living 53 years, you would think someone wonders how you are doing. Days go by, then months and years of time where there is never a voice saying "I wonder how old Dave is doing". What have I done to drive everyone away from me?

Can someone really survive living without a connection

to another human being? I mean who would want to live in a world without connection to anyone? What have I possibly done to be put on this island of loneliness? For a person that has so much love to give I just don't understand why there is no one out there for me.

ADDICTION

How could she do this to me, lead me to a way of life that is so painful but also full of such pleasure. These two things are never seen by the outside world but have a huge effect on all things that come into contact with them. At times I think how she could pass this addiction to her child knowing the effect it can have on me. To spend endless amount of time and energy making sure there is no chance of not passing along the addiction. To put this burden in place no matter the cost.

Some would say that she has wasted her time passing along something that not many people find a value in any more. As a young child, it is very hard to understand why she would do this to me knowing how it will make me different. In life there are many things that don't make sense to you until you have lived a long life.

This addiction is called responsibility. To impose this affliction on another person is a great gift and a great pain at the same time. Responsibility seems to be a quality that you see less and less of every day. Although having this addiction can sometimes be very painful and full of frustration, it is also one of the greatest gifts my mother could have given me.

In a world of people that refuse to take the blame for their mistakes I'm so happy that I was given the backbone to say,

"I'm sorry that was my mistake and I will do whatever it takes to correct my error". There are so many people out there that will do whatever it takes to pass the blame to someone else no matter how much it may hurt the other person. I think that one of the greatest feelings in life is just to say" hey that was me and I'm sorry about that, I will try to make the right steps to not let it happen again".

There is no way you can grow if you are afraid to stand up and say "I'm not perfect but I will keep trying to do my best". So I want to take this time to thank that wonderful woman that made sure the addiction of responsibility was passed along to me. The reason I call it an addiction is because the more you do it the better it makes you feel inside. No one can see that place inside of you that glows with pride. There is no prize awarded for being responsible that anyone can see, it's just something that is there because that's just who you are.

NO NIGHTMARES!

Some people might think that not having any nightmares would be a blessing in life. I think I would believe it to be a blessing as well if it were not for the fact that I have no recollection of any nightmares in my life. You see in my world it's so hard to fall asleep at night... knowing that you're living in a nightmare to begin with.

There's a small chance that I might have some nightmares from time to time. I never remember them because on most times I am waking up to something that is much worse, the ongoing nightmare that is Jordyn's life. There is no way to count the number of nights that I have been awakened by the cries of my daughter in pain, nor can I count the number of nights where sleeping is just not an option. Nobody will ever know the amount of praying, wishing or just plain begging I have done in an attempt to just have the pain go away for just a week.

Every morning I get up I try to put on my best positive face for the world to see. Man it's getting harder and harder to pull off that trick these days! I've always been a person who tries to look on the positive side of life, but how many times does the world think I can get up in the morning and dig through a giant pile of shit to find my silver lining for that day. Not to mention my poor daughter's feelings about this life that was forced upon her. Finding the energy to battle on against the pain monster is a task that gets harder by the day. Jordyn and I have managed to carry on this war for more than 10 years now. Even soldiers get to have a little R&R when they are at war.

I'm just so very worried about my little girl. She really seems to be on her last leg and I don't know how strong that leg was to begin with. Let's not forget about the real scary part of this nightmare and that would be Mr. HIV/AIDS living in Jordyn's backseat. That's a nightmare no one wants to wake up to.

LAST DAYS

Well today I went to visit my oldest friend I've had outside of my family. The reason for the visit was not a happy one.

My friend, Andy, was my high school sweetheart and the longest friendship I have ever had. Over the years she built a strong relationship with my daughter as well. These last days have been very hard on my daughter, because over the years of her short life she has lost too many friends already.

We came to visit her because she has been very sick for a long time now; nobody really knows how long she will last.

It's a really weird place to be in because I think we are both thinking to ourselves, "Will this be the last time we see each other?" Neither one of us wants to say it out loud. I mean if you were going to say something what would it be? She's at a point in life her where she doesn't really cares about living to battle on against all these medical issues that lie ahead of her. At what point do you just say "fuck all the struggling to only struggle another day?" How many times can a person be challenged before the challenges start to tear you down instead of build you up. I know in my world I have gotten to the point where I ask myself that question more and more every day.

You know when I walk into the hospital tomorrow, we both know it could be for the last time. Knowing that what the hell do you talk about, surely not the future. This could be a very scary topic for all. You break down and cry, saying goodbye in a way that leaves options open, could she have a miracle turnaround.

What are the last words you should say? I really don't know, but a guess I will come up with something good to say before I walk out the door tomorrow on my way back to Colorado. I know one thing she will always be my friend and I will always have her in my heart.

STRONG ENOUGH

Am I strong enough? That is a question I've been asking myself lately. You know the saying "God only gives you what you are strong enough to handle". Over the last 26 years there have been many challenging times that I have managed to live through one way or another.

This time I feel like the challenge in front of me is going to consume me in many ways. I never thought after all I've been through I would end up in such a place. I was always told that if you worked hard that in the end you would reap the rewards of your hard work, well that is not at all where I am now. After busting my ass and giving everything I had to my career. The reward was having to start over in my career in a sense. I now have to learn all new areas of our business that are not my forte. I wonder if my body and my mind will have the strength or desire to learn this new way of life. I guess like with all the other challenges I have face in my life, I will

Find a way to overcome this obstacle in a positive way.

CHAPTER 5

THE MIRACLE OF BECOMING AN ADULT

DEAR SISTER,

I just want to let you know how much having you in my life has meant to me. It has been a long road to be on the last 18 years, but at least I have had you and DJ riding shotgun for me. That's why I always walk out into the world trying not bringing the problems with me. It is because of your support that I always try to put my best foot forward when it comes to DJensen Electrics. I'm proud to be working for you guys. I also cherish all that I have learned from the both of you along the way.

I know that things right now are not the best of times for Jordyn and I. I know she has hurt you as well as others. I know that she has made some terrible choices & that reflects on her as a person. It really hurt me to hear you say that you feel like you've wasted the last 18 years of your life due to Jordyn's actions. I don't think we should let such a small moment in time erase all the good things that she has done. She is a young person having to live with HIV. I don't excuse her behavior and I've been trying to figure out a way to get through to her. Right now I don't think Jordyn even knows who Jordyn is.

You know she's never murdered anyone, stolen a car and she's not a terrorist. Well maybe on some of her really bad days she may seem like a terrorist.

You know I've had my days dealing with Jordyn myself and it's so easy to let the anger take ahold of you because you feel you have been hurt and you want strike back. I have definitely learned over the years that when life is driving you insane, it's really hard to remain calm. I have definitely learned over the years that in these times of insanity and anger it is definitely a lot safer for everyone involved if I just sit down and let the dust settle before I take any action.

Once I'm in a calmer place, it's much easier for me to look at the situation and try to figure out how I can help my daughter return to her normal self, as well as for her to control her emotions in the future, and make the right decisions.

The reason I am writing you this letter is to say thank you for starters, and to tell you I love you and hate to see you hold all that anger inside of you. You know if I hadn't found a way to get rid of the anger in my life and all of the frustration that I have lived through over the past 18 years, I would probably be dead right now.

Sometimes it takes a lot of work for me to de-fuse myself, but I feel like I keep getting better at it every day. I guess since I just don't like seeing people I love that upset, as well as holding onto all of that stress and anger longer than they need to. When it's in the past, we can no longer do anything about it, except to try and find the lesson in these rough times we have had to live through. I know going through these times for Jordyn and, myself I have asked myself does Jordyn really love me? How could she treat me like this? In the end you know she truly loves you Johanna. She is just a kid growing up making mistakes the way we all did when we were her age.

You're such a wonderful sister, and not a person who gives in very quickly, take a deep breath and get back in the game!

Love, Your baby brother.

BEING IN THE WRONG!

The most upsetting thing about being a parent is when your child has done something wrong. We all know that no one is perfect and that making mistakes is how we are supposed to learn in life.

No parent wants to hear from someone else that their child is being bad, that information coming from someone outside of your family is a tough thing to choke down.

Well, when it's your closest family member telling you how horrible your child has been, it just makes it that much harder to choke down. The first thing you want to do is defend your child, but know you can't really go there when you have been an eye witness to the hand in the crime.

The really hard part is that you want to make things right. Only at this point that's not a possibility. The thing is no matter how hard you try smooth things over to get things back to normal, it is not in your power. This just leaves the parent wondering how we will ever be able to put this family back together. Well if this was a young child, he would just take a little bit to be forgiven, but when that child is an adult of 24 and has gone to the well one too many times... forgiveness it is not so easy to find.

Boy do I wish there were some magic spell that could make

this time in life just disappear. I have had to live through a lot of challenges over the past 20 years but this one really hurts the most.

Hearing the pain and disappointment in my sister's voice just makes my stomach turn inside out. I worked so hard over the years to not let them down after all they had done for me, yet a letdown is what they got even if it did not come directly from me. It did come from my home. Day after day I sit and think it's not like she wasn't taught about not doing these things she did. In my daughter's defense she says she will pay back all that was taken without asking, but can she really pay back for all of the pain and disappointment she has inflicted on Johanna and DJ? They are the greatest people I know in this world and it kills me deep down in my soul every time I think about what my daughter has done. I guess the only thing that's going to heal this wound is plenty of time and my daughter living up her word by paying back the money. Whether she wants to think about it or not there is a deep scar that is dividing are too little worlds right now and she is the one that made that scar. Whether it was out of malice or not, the scar is still there needing some TLC before it can begin to heal.

I'll be the first one to take a step forward to start the healing, but I'm pretty sure I will be standing there alone for quite a long time.

GOING INTO ADULTHOOD

Dear Jordyn,

Well Jordan today is the big day. Today you start one of the biggest journeys you have ever been on. Today you truly become an adult. No matter what anybody says to you, you can tell them that on this day you decided to change the course of your life forever. On this day you decided to make a change in the direction your life would be going. You made this decision in spite of the fact that it scared you to the point of tears. On this day you were adult enough to stand up for yourself & say "I can do this".

There have been many proud moments that you have given me. Many, many times you have shown me what a brave girl you are. Well this day tops them all for me. I know you're nervous and scared, I also know how strong you can be. You by far are the strongest person I've ever known... every day you have shown your strength to me. Every day that you have not given up has only made you stronger and more prepared for this challenge.

As for this new challenge I hope you can jump in all the way up to your head, completely giving yourself to this program that could possibly change your life forever.... If you let it.

Please open your mind and your heart to all the new things that will be laid at your feet. Not many people get the opportunity to change the direction of their life. So please take it all in and make the best of this time. You will have time to yourself to really get to know who Jordyn Driver really is, and who she really wants to be.

There will be no one there to cloud your mind with what they think Jordyn Driver should be. This is your time to discover who you really are deep down inside. This is your time to find the light that shines inside of you. This is your time to tell the world hey this is who I am… like me or not… this is who I am for the good, the bad and the ugly.

You've always been a shining star in my life and I know that you will continue to shine throughout this time. When you walk out those doors at the end of your quests, you will be shining even brighter than today.

Jordyn, you will always be my hero. You will always be my source of energy, and last but not least, you will always be my sunshine, my only sunshine, you make me happy when skies are gray, you are my sunshine my only sunshine so please don't take my sunshine away.

I love you Jordyn,

Love Maddy

A NEW ERA?

I suppose you would say that my little Jordyn has started a new era in life. I guess I will have to take you back five or six days. That is when Jordyn and I had our last argument as father and child. Well one thing led to another and in the end Jordyn was no longer welcome at home, that is until she learned to respect the house as well as her father. There were two choices, one being respectful while living in our home, the other live on your friend's couches. Well to my surprise Jordyn decided to choose surfing couches instead of coming home. She says to me "Dad it's just time," like I'm the clueless one. Man how our children can make us laugh as well as cry in the same moment.

I really don't know where we will go from here, but I'm sure that will be another story somewhere down the road for sure.

DEAR CEDAR

Dear Cedar scholarship committee,

The first thing I'd like to say, is never my life did I think that I would be in this situation that I am in today especially after surviving HIV/AIDS for the last 23 years. My motivation for wanting to rehabilitate myself is that I have not battled HIV/AIDS for the last 23 years of my life to let these drugs take over who I really am.

For the last 6 ½ years I've been struggling with an abdominal pain that seems to be invisible to diagnose, but very visible when it comes to the pain I feel day in and day out. In the beginning my stomach pain came from only one spot in my body, but now my Dad and I, as well as all of my medical team, feel that a lot of this pain is coming from the side effects of years of having to use pain meds to bring the pain back down to a level that I could live with.

As a result of the battle I have waged against the stomach pain, I have also built up a dependency on pain meds I was prescribed by the pain clinic and the ones I received at many of my ER trips we took in the middle of the night to subdue the pain. As a result I am not the person I feel I used to be. My energy level and my ability to focus have both suffered immensely. I've also noticed that I have developed many different mood changes at the drop of a hat, which has caused a lot of conflict with my family. Also the lack of energy and focus has made it very difficult to attend school or hold a job.

Overall I feel that getting back to a clean slate in life can only help me to reconnect with the world around me as well as with my family and friends whom I have been alienated during this period of my life.

I know this process will not be easy, but I feel there are just too many positives reasons to succeed with the treatment and also follow through and stay on a path that puts me where I really want to be. After all I haven't survived all these crappy health issues to give up now.

Thank you very much for your consideration.

THE COST OF LOSING JORDYN

Yeah that's what it says the cost of losing Jordyn, because no matter how we got here or whose fault it is, the fact remains the same. Somehow along the way we lost the girl we knew as Jordyn. You see the thing is, no one saw her disappear, I just looked up one day and thought, "Who the hell is that that girl sitting on the couch?" I don't ever remember meeting her, and to tell you the truth, I don't think I really care for her that much. Just looking at her I can tell she's got an attitude problem. Then I thought wait a minute you can't just label her like that. You better give her a little more time before you cast your opinion on her.

Well my dear Jordyn, if I were to attach a cost to this whole pain med issue, it would be the cost of losing you. Because in all honesty I feel that a lot of ways you let yourself down and by doing so you lost that wonderful girl that I knew and loved so dearly. Somewhere in the 6 ½ of your battle you stopping being you (that would be the girl who never knew what it was like to let being sick control any part of our world) and started becoming a person that I liked less and less as the battle waged on. Living with this new girl got harder and harder because the fight just was not there, like in the days of old Jordyn. In the old days I never questioned whether you tried this remedy or tried that remedy, because you were always trying to get out of being sick so you could go outside and play.

I think the biggest cost you could have put in my lap is that I had to doubt you on many occasions. That was something I thought I would never have to do, because before you could even talk we always had one thing between us and that was trust. Those pain killers came in and sold your trust to the highest bidder without you even knowing it. That's where the true evil lies in those damn painkillers. While you are down and in pain, those painkillers are like a friendly handheld out to you. You not knowing what you're doing you take the help and began thinking wow that is really nice of them to help me. What you didn't really know was, what a trap it really was for you.

So as you look back on this whole experience, I would give you this one really good piece of advice, no matter what it is, drugs, religion or collecting bottle caps. If what you are doing in life makes you into somebody you do not recognize. Maybe you have to step back from whatever it is you are doing, and realize that this thing is not who you are and you need to walk away from it and back to the person you knew in the beginning.

My dear Jordyn, I know you will find a way because deep down inside you are that wonderful lady I love so much and could not be any prouder of if I tried.

Love Maddy

AFTERWORD

Well here you are at the end of this very unconventional book. I know that you may have many questions after reading my book. Well even after all these years, so do I. So many things have happened over the past 26 years it is really hard for me to put them in any real order.

After living a life of always being the counter puncher, I feel pretty punch drunk on some days when, I try to remember it all. That is why the book ended up the way it did - small snapshots of time. In some ways I think that was the only way I could handle it back then.

You know living through the last 26 years has really been quite the roll-a-coaster at times and has challenged me at every turn along the way. I do feel like I have learned a great deal. I have learned to never worry about a problem until it is really a problem. I have learned to find the silver lining no matter how impossible it may seem to find at the time. I have learned how to laugh even when I want to cry, and how I have learned how to find a way to always make my little girl smile. I have learned to never let the problems I may be facing become a reason to lash out at the people around me. I have learned how to sit quietly and think before I react (well maybe not always) to a situation. Last but not least, I have learned the hard way just what a person can live through and then have the strength to do it all over again and again.

In the end I feel very lucky to have learned all of the things I have over the past 26 years, because it will help me to continue with this life that still has many more stories to tell.

ACKNOWLEDGEMENTS

Well it is at this time I want to acknowledge the people that were very instrumental in my survival over the past 26 years. First and foremost are the wonderful angels that have been in my corner since the very beginning, I call them my family. To the most wonderful Mother anyone could have. What can I say to let the world know what an incredible Mother and Father she has been in my life; There are no amount of words that can say what a blessing it was to have you in my corner all of these years. No one could ever replace her. As for my Dad, well you also handled that for me as well Mom, because that other guy was just never there when I needed him.

To Johanna and DJ - wow what an anchor you two have

been for me. You have been my support in so many ways. Johanna, you have been that hard ass sister that would never let me quit, as well as that sister with the biggest heart when I really needed a hug. Always being there in my corner no matter how insane things would get in my world.

DJ, if I ever had the chance to pick a father or a brother you would be my choice every day and twice on Sunday. To have you in my life has been a true gift from the heavens. From all of the things you have taught me and all of the times you have been there for me time and time again, there are not enough words to say how lucky I am that you married my sister.

Between the two of you I always found a way to battle on no matter how crazy things got, because I knew you were there for us. Having you in my corner helped me to find the energy to carry on. You are truly my guardian angels.

To Michelle and Steve in -spite of all your own medical nightmares you both always found a way to let me know things would be alright. I could always count on some really sound advice and comforting phone calls right when I really needed it.

I also want to thank all of the people who have prayed for us and thought good thoughts for Jordyn and our family. You were all a great source of hope and energy that help us battle on in ways we will never know. For all of you that held on to Jordyn's prayer pins for many years I will never be able to thank you enough!

Last but not least, my wonderful daughter Jordyn. I truly feel lucky to be your Maddy. Like I have said to you many times, before you are the strongest and bravest person I have ever known. You have been since day one my purest source of energy. Watching you grow up doing all you had to do to survive without ever complaining along the way was my greatest pleasure. If someone were to ask me if I were to do it all over again, I would never change one single day that I had with you. YOU HAVE ALWAYS BEEN MY SUNSHINE.

Printed in the United States
By Bookmasters